Occipital Neuralgia

A Beginner's Guide and Overview to Managing the Condition through Diet, with Sample Curated Recipes

mf

copyright © 2022 Patrick Marshwell

All rights reserved No part of this book may be reproduced, or stored in a retrieval system, or transmitted in any form or by any means, electronic, mechanical, photocopying, recording, or otherwise, without express written permission of the publisher.

Disclaimer

By reading this disclaimer, you are accepting the terms of the disclaimer in full. If you disagree with this disclaimer, please do not read the guide.

All of the content within this guide is provided for informational and educational purposes only, and should not be accepted as independent medical or other professional advice. The author is not a doctor, physician, nurse, mental health provider, or registered nutritionist/dietician. Therefore, using and reading this guide does not establish any form of a physician-patient relationship.

Always consult with a physician or another qualified health provider with any issues or questions you might have regarding any sort of medical condition. Do not ever disregard any qualified professional medical advice or delay seeking that advice because of anything you have read in this guide. The information in this guide is not intended to be any sort of medical advice and should not be used in lieu of any medical advice by a licensed and qualified medical professional.

The information in this guide has been compiled from a variety of known sources. However, the author cannot attest to or guarantee the accuracy of each source and thus should not be held liable for any errors or omissions.

You acknowledge that the publisher of this guide will not be held liable for any loss or damage of any kind incurred as a result of this guide or the reliance on any information provided within this guide. You acknowledge and agree that you assume all risk and responsibility for any action you undertake in response to the information in this guide.

Using this guide does not guarantee any particular result (e.g., weight loss or a cure). By reading this guide, you acknowledge that there are no guarantees to any specific outcome or results you can expect.

All product names, diet plans, or names used in this guide are for identification purposes only and are the property of their respective owners. The use of these names does not imply endorsement. All other trademarks cited herein are the property of their respective owners.

Where applicable, this guide is not intended to be a substitute for the original work of this diet plan and is, at most, a supplement to the original work for this diet plan and never a direct substitute. This guide is a personal expression of the facts of that diet plan.

Where applicable, persons shown in the cover images are stock photography models and the publisher has obtained the rights to use the images through license agreements with third-party stock image companies.

Table of Contents

Introduction   7
What Is Occipital Neuralgia?   10
    What Causes Occipital Neuralgia?   10
    Occipital Neuralgia Symptoms   12
    When to see a doctor?   13
    Diagnosing Occipital Neuralgia   14
    Medical Treatments for Occipital Neuralgia   15
    What are the home remedies for occipital neuralgia?   17
    Managing Occipital Neuralgia Through Home Remedies and Natural Methods   20
Managing Occipital Neuralgia Through Diet and Nutrition   23
    Principles of Anti-Inflammatory Diet for Occipital Neuralgia 23
    Benefits of an Anti-Inflammatory Diet for Occipital Neuralgia 27
    Disadvantages of the Diet   29
5-Step-by-Step Guide to Starting an Anti-Inflammatory Diet for Occipital Neuralgia   31
    Step 1: Educate Yourself   31
    Step 2: Eliminate Inflammatory Foods   33
    Step 3: Plan Balanced Meals   36
    Step 4: Stay Hydrated   40
    Step 5: Monitor and Adjust   42
    Foods to Eat   44
    Foods to Avoid   47
    Practical Tips for Avoiding Inflammatory Foods   50
7-Day Sample Meal Plan   52
Sample Recipes   57
    Baked Flounder   58
    Baked Salmon   59
    Lemon-Baked Salmon   60

Cod Pea Curry	62
Grilled Tuna	64
Baked Sea Bass and Lemon Dressing	65
Roasted Bone Broth	66
Salmon Fillet with Lemon and Garlic	68
Cauliflower Rice with Chicken and Broccoli	70
Slow Cooker Dairy-Free Buttered Chicken	71
Ginger Chicken Stir Fry	73
Cheddar Turkey Deviled Egg	75
Conclusion	**77**
FAQs	**80**
References and Helpful Links	**83**

Introduction

Occipital neuralgia can be a debilitating condition, causing intense stabbing or electric-shock-like pain in the upper neck, back of the head, and behind the ears. Often mistaken for migraines or other types of headaches, occipital neuralgia is a distinct neurological disorder that stems from irritation or injury to the occipital nerves. Understanding this difference is crucial for effective management.

To effectively manage occipital neuralgia, one must first grasp the root causes and recognize the symptoms. The occipital nerves run from the top of the spinal cord to the scalp, and any compression, inflammation, or trauma to these nerves can result in severe discomfort. Awareness of this condition is essential for seeking appropriate medical attention and exploring various therapeutic options.

This guide aims to shed light on the latest advancements and holistic approaches to managing occipital neuralgia. From conventional treatments to lifestyle modifications and innovative therapies, the guide offers a comprehensive roadmap for those navigating this challenging condition.

Living with occipital neuralgia can be challenging, but it doesn't have to be a life sentence of pain. Effective management begins with accurate diagnosis and tailored treatment plans. Beyond immediate relief, long-term strategies are vital for regaining control over one's life and enhancing overall well-being.

Discover a range of management techniques that go beyond medication, including physical therapy, stress management, and cutting-edge treatments. This guide covers a variety of methodologies designed to offer hope and tangible relief for those suffering from occipital neuralgia.

In this beginner's guide, we'll provide an in-depth discussion of the following:

- What is Occipital Neuralgia?
- What causes occipital neuralgia?
- What are the symptoms of occipital neuralgia?
- When to see a doctor?
- How is occipital neuralgia diagnosed?
- What are the medical treatments for occipital neuralgia?
- How to prevent occipital neuralgia?
- How to manage occipital neuralgia through home remedies and natural methods?
- Managing occipital neuralgia through diet and nutrition.

Effectively managing occipital neuralgia necessitates a proactive strategy. This guide is a comprehensive resource, providing valuable insights and practical advice for those seeking relief. By delving into various treatments and preventive measures, individuals can make well-informed decisions and take control of their health. For anyone dealing with occipital neuralgia, this guide offers the essential information needed to understand and manage the condition more effectively.

What Is Occipital Neuralgia?

Occipital neuralgia is a neurological condition that causes sharp, shooting pain in the back of the head, neck, and behind the eyes. It occurs when the occipital nerves – located at the base of the skull – become inflamed or injured.

The intense pain experienced with occipital neuralgia can be debilitating, affecting one's ability to work, perform daily activities, and enjoy life. The condition may also lead to feelings of isolation and frustration due to its impact on quality of life.

What Causes Occipital Neuralgia?

Several different factors can contribute to the development of occipital neuralgia. In some cases, the underlying cause is unknown. However, some of the more common causes include:

Pinched nerves

Occipital neuralgia is a condition that causes intense, throbbing pain in the back of the head and neck. The pain is caused by compression or damage to the occipital nerves, which are responsible for transmitting signals from the back of the head to the brain. In most cases, the underlying cause of occipital neuralgia is a pinched nerve. This can occur due to muscle tension, repetitive motion, poor posture, injury, or inflammation.

Muscular strain

Muscular strain is one of the most common causes of occipital neuralgia. The muscles in the back of the head and neck are constantly being used to support the weight of the head. When these muscles become strained or tight, they can put pressure on the nerves that run through them.

This can lead to pain in the upper neck and back of the head. Physical therapy can often help to relieve muscular strain and prevent it from recurring.

Injury

Occipital neuralgia is a type of headache that is caused by injury to the occipital nerves. These nerves are located at the back of the head and run from the base of the skull to the top of the neck. Injury to these nerves can occur due to a variety of reasons, including car accidents, sports injuries, and surgery.

Tumor

Tumors can put pressure on the nerves in the back of the head, causing pain and inflammation. In some cases, tumors can also cause the nerves to become stretched or damaged. This can lead to several symptoms, including headaches, neck pain, and sensitivity to light.

These are just a few potential causes of occipital neuralgia, and it's important to speak with a healthcare professional for an accurate diagnosis and treatment plan. In some cases, the underlying cause may be unknown or difficult to determine.

Occipital Neuralgia Symptoms

Most people have never heard of occipital neuralgia, a condition that causes pain in the back of the head. This type of neuralgia is a result of damage or irritation to the occipital nerve, which runs from the base of the skull to the muscles in the back of the head. The symptoms of this condition can be very severe and include throbbing or burning pain, sensitivity to light, and nausea.

- *Pain*: The most common symptom of occipital neuralgia is pain that begins at the base of the skull and radiates upward toward the scalp. This pain can be aching, searing, or throbbing in nature, and is often made worse by movement.
- *Headache*: Occipital neuralgia is a condition that causes headaches. The pain typically occurs on one or both sides of the head, and it can range from mild to severe.

- ***Sensitivity to light***: Many people who have occipital neuralgia also find that they are sensitive to light. This sensitivity can make it difficult to be in well-lit areas or to look at bright screens, such as computers or TVs.
- ***Nausea***: Nausea is another common symptom of occipital neuralgia. This nausea can be so severe that it leads to vomiting.
- ***Difficulty in concentrating***: The pain and other symptoms of occipital neuralgia can make it difficult to concentrate on tasks. This can lead to problems at work or school.

If you experience any of these symptoms, it is important to see a doctor for diagnosis and treatment. If left untreated, occipital neuralgia can lead to chronic pain and disability.

When to see a doctor?

If you are experiencing any of the signs and symptoms of occipital neuralgia, you should get medical assistance as soon as possible. This holds in particular if the pain is severe or if it prevents you from partaking in activities that are typically a part of your daily routine.

If you see a medical professional, he or she will be able to diagnose you with occipital neuralgia and devise a treatment plan that will assist in reducing the severity of the symptoms you are experiencing.

Diagnosing Occipital Neuralgia

If you think you may be suffering from occipital neuralgia, it's important to see a doctor for an accurate diagnosis. Your doctor will likely ask about your medical history and symptoms and perform a physical exam. They may also order tests like MRI or CT scans to rule out other conditions with similar symptoms, such as migraines or tension headaches.

1. *Medical History*: Your doctor will want to know about your medical history, including any previous injuries or illnesses that may be relevant. He or she will also ask about your family's medical history to see if there is a genetic component to your condition.
2. *Symptoms*: Be sure to tell your doctor all of the symptoms you are experiencing, even if they seem unrelated. This information will help your doctor make an accurate diagnosis.
3. *Physical Exam*: Your doctor will perform a physical exam, during which he or she will check for areas of tenderness in your neck and head. He or she may also order tests, such as MRI or CT scans, to rule out other conditions with similar symptoms.
4. *MRI or CT Scans*: These imaging tests can help your doctor rule out other conditions, such as migraines or tension headaches, that may be causing your symptoms.

Once your doctor has made a diagnosis of occipital neuralgia, he or she will work with you to develop a treatment plan.

Medical Treatments for Occipital Neuralgia

There is no one-size-fits-all treatment for occipital neuralgia; instead, your doctor will work with you to develop a treatment plan that meets your unique needs. Common treatments for occipital neuralgia include over-the-counter pain relievers, physical therapy, epidural injections, and steroid injections. In some cases, surgery may be necessary to relieve pressure on the affected nerves.

Pain relievers

Over-the-counter pain relievers, such as ibuprofen or acetaminophen, can help to relieve the pain of occipital neuralgia. Ibuprofen is a nonsteroidal anti-inflammatory drug (NSAID) that can reduce inflammation and pain. Acetaminophen is a less potent pain reliever that is often used in conjunction with other pain relievers. Both drugs are available over the counter and can be taken orally or applied topically.

Tricyclic antidepressants

These drugs work by inhibiting the reuptake of certain neurotransmitters, which helps to reduce pain signals. In addition, tricyclic antidepressants can also help to reduce inflammation and relax muscles. As a result, they can provide significant relief for people who suffer from occipital neuralgia. If you are considering treatment for this condition, be sure to discuss the pros and cons of tricyclic antidepressants with your doctor.

Anticonvulsants

Anticonvulsants are a type of medication that is typically used to treat seizures. However, they can also be effective in treating other conditions, such as occipital neuralgia. Anticonvulsants work by reducing the amount of nerve activity in the brain. This can help to relieve pressure and pain in the back of the head. A doctor may prescribe an anticonvulsant for a short period to relieve symptoms or for long-term treatment.

Epidural injections

Epidural injections are a type of treatment used to relieve pain in the neck, back, and legs. The injections are most often given to people who have herniated disks or other conditions that put pressure on the nerves.

The goal of epidural injections is to reduce inflammation and pain by delivering medication directly to the affected area. Several different types of medication can be used for epidural injections, but steroids are the most common.

Steroids work by reducing inflammation, which can help to relieve pain and improve function. Epidural injections are typically given on an outpatient basis, and most people experience significant relief after just a few treatments.

Radiofrequency ablation

This involves using heat to destroy the nerve tissue. The procedure is typically performed under local anesthesia, and it typically takes about 30 minutes to complete. Radiofrequency ablation is generally considered to be safe and effective, but it is important to discuss all of your options with a qualified healthcare provider before making any decisions.

Surgery

Surgery is rarely needed to treat occipital neuralgia. However, if the condition is caused by a tumor or compression of the nerve, surgery may be necessary to relieve the pressure on the nerve.

Be sure to consult with your doctor before beginning any new treatment, as some treatments may not be appropriate for all people. Treatment for occipital neuralgia should be tailored to the individual patient, taking into account the severity of the pain and the side effects of the medication.

What are the home remedies for occipital neuralgia?

Managing occipital neuralgia at home can complement medical treatments and help alleviate symptoms. Here are some effective home remedies to consider:

Cold and Heat Therapy

Applying cold packs or heat pads to the affected area can provide significant relief. Cold packs help reduce inflammation and numb sharp pain, while heat pads can relax tight muscles and improve blood flow.

Gentle Neck Exercises

Stretching and strengthening exercises for the neck can help relieve tension in the occipital region. Gentle yoga poses, such as neck stretches and shoulder rolls, may also be beneficial. Always perform these exercises slowly and avoid any movements that exacerbate your pain.

Massage

Regularly massaging the neck and upper back can reduce muscle tension and improve blood circulation. You can use your hands or a massage tool to gently knead the muscles around the occipital nerves.

Over-the-Counter Pain Relievers

Non-prescription pain relievers like ibuprofen or acetaminophen can help manage mild to moderate pain. Be sure to follow the recommended dosage instructions on the packaging or consult your healthcare provider.

Relaxation Techniques

Stress often exacerbates occipital neuralgia. Incorporating relaxation techniques such as deep breathing exercises, meditation, or mindfulness can help manage stress and reduce pain frequency.

Hydration and Diet

Staying well-hydrated and maintaining a balanced diet can support overall nerve health. Foods rich in omega-3 fatty acids, antioxidants, and vitamins B12 and D may be particularly beneficial.

Proper Posture

Maintaining good posture, especially during activities like working at a computer or reading, can reduce strain on the neck and occipital nerves. Ergonomic adjustments to your workspace can also be helpful.

Sleep Hygiene

Ensuring good sleep hygiene by using a supportive pillow and maintaining a proper sleeping position can help reduce neck strain. Aim for a consistent sleep schedule and create a restful environment.

While these home remedies can offer relief, they should be used in conjunction with professional medical advice. Always consult with a healthcare provider before starting any new treatment regimen for occipital neuralgia.

Managing Occipital Neuralgia Through Home Remedies and Natural Methods

There are a few natural methods that can help you manage the pain and symptoms of occipital neuralgia. Some of these methods include:

Ice and Heat Packs

Ice and heat packs can help to alleviate the pain and discomfort associated with this condition. Ice packs can be applied for 15-20 minutes at a time, several times a day. This will help to numb the area and reduce inflammation.

Heat packs can also be used, but should be applied for shorter periods (5-10 minutes). The heat helps to increase blood flow to the area, which can aid in the healing process. While both ice and heat packs can provide relief, it is important to consult with a doctor before using either treatment.

Neck Exercises

Neck exercises are a simple, effective way to relieve the pain of occipital neuralgia. By gently stretching and strengthening the muscles in the back of the neck, these exercises can help to take pressure off of the Occipital nerves. In addition, neck exercises can also help to improve the range of motion and prevent further injury.

For best results, it is recommended to perform these exercises daily. However, if you experience any pain or discomfort, be sure to stop immediately and consult your doctor.

Massage

Occipital neuralgia is a condition that results in pain in the back of the head and neck. Massage is one of the most effective home remedies for this condition. It helps to loosen tight muscles and relieve tension headaches.

For the best results, use a light, circular motion. Start at the base of the skull and work your way up to the temples. You can also use your fingers to massage the muscles on either side of the spine. Be sure to drink plenty of water after your massage to help flush out toxins.

Acupuncture

Acupuncture is a traditional Chinese medicine technique that involves inserting thin needles into the skin at specific points on the body. Acupuncture is thought to stimulate the release of pain-relieving chemicals in the body and can help to reduce the pain of occipital neuralgia.

Herbal Remedies

Some herbal remedies may help to reduce inflammation and pain. For example, ginger has been shown to have anti-inflammatory properties, and it has been used to treat various conditions such as arthritis. Similarly, turmeric contains a compound called curcumin, which has also been shown to have anti-inflammatory effects. Thus, these herbs may help to reduce pain and inflammation associated with occipital neuralgia.

Diet

Eating a healthy diet that includes plenty of fruits, vegetables, and whole grains can help to reduce inflammation and pain.

Chiropractic Care

When the bones of the spine are out of alignment, it can cause several problems, including pain, reduced mobility, and numbness. Chiropractic care is a treatment that aims to correct these issues by realigning the spine. This can provide relief from conditions like occipital neuralgia, which is characterized by pain and pressure in the nerves of the head and neck. In addition to relieving pain, chiropractic care can also help to improve the range of motion and reduce inflammation.

Be sure to consult with your doctor before beginning any new home treatment, as some treatments may not be appropriate for all people.

Managing Occipital Neuralgia Through Diet and Nutrition

In addition to conventional treatments like those mentioned above, there are several things you can do at home to manage your pain and improve your quality of life. One of the most important things you can do is pay attention to your diet and nutrition.

Eating a healthy diet rich in fruits, vegetables, whole grains, and lean protein can help reduce inflammation throughout your body and ease nerve pain. Additionally, drinking plenty of water each day will help keep your body hydrated and may also help reduce inflammation. Finally, avoid triggers like caffeine and alcohol that can exacerbate nerve pain.

Principles of Anti-Inflammatory Diet for Occipital Neuralgia

Diet plays a crucial role in managing occipital neuralgia by supporting overall nerve health and reducing inflammation. Here are the key principles to follow for an occipital neuralgia-friendly diet:

1. **Anti-Inflammatory Foods**

   Incorporate foods that have anti-inflammatory properties to help reduce nerve irritation and pain. These include:

   - Fruits and Vegetables: Especially those rich in antioxidants, such as berries, leafy greens, tomatoes, and bell peppers.
   - Healthy Fats: Sources like olive oil, avocados, and nuts.
   - Omega-3 Fatty Acids: Found in fatty fish (like salmon and mackerel), flaxseeds, and chia seeds.

2. **Magnesium-Rich Foods**

   Magnesium is known to support nerve function and may help alleviate muscle tension and spasms. Include:

   - Dark Leafy Greens: Spinach, kale, and Swiss chard.
   - Nuts and Seeds: Almonds, sunflower seeds, and pumpkin seeds.
   - Whole Grains: Brown rice, quinoa, and oats.

3. **Adequate Hydration**

   Staying hydrated is essential for overall health and can help prevent muscle stiffness and tension. Aim to drink at least 8 glasses of water daily, and consider hydrating foods such as:

- Water-Rich Fruits: Watermelon, cucumber, and oranges.
- Herbal Teas: Chamomile, peppermint, or ginger tea.

4. **Vitamin B12**

Vitamin B12 is vital for nerve health. Ensure you include:

- Animal Products: Lean meats, fish, eggs, and dairy products.
- Fortified Foods: Cereals and plant-based milk alternatives.

5. **Vitamin D**

Vitamin D deficiency can affect nerve function and pain levels. Sources include:

- Fatty Fish: Salmon, mackerel, and tuna.
- Fortified Foods: Dairy products, orange juice, and cereals.
- Sun Exposure: Moderate sunlight exposure can help the body synthesize vitamin D naturally.

6. **Avoid Trigger Foods**

Certain foods might exacerbate inflammation or trigger headaches. Common culprits to avoid include:

- Processed Foods: High in unhealthy fats and additives.

- Sugary Foods and Beverages: Excessive sugar intake can lead to inflammation.
- Alcohol and Caffeine: Can dehydrate and potentially trigger symptoms.

7. **Balanced Meals**

   Consuming balanced meals throughout the day helps maintain stable blood sugar levels, which can prevent headache triggers. Focus on:

   - Lean Proteins: Chicken, turkey, tofu, and legumes.
   - Complex Carbohydrates: Whole grains, sweet potatoes, and legumes.
   - Healthy Fats: Avocado, nuts, and seeds.

8. **Regular Meals**

   Skipping meals can lead to blood sugar fluctuations, potentially triggering headache symptoms. Try to eat small, balanced meals regularly to maintain energy levels.

By following these dietary principles, individuals with occipital neuralgia can support their overall health and potentially reduce the frequency and severity of their symptoms. Always consult with a healthcare provider or nutritionist to tailor a diet plan to your specific needs and circumstances.

Benefits of an Anti-Inflammatory Diet for Occipital Neuralgia

Adopting an anti-inflammatory diet can offer significant advantages for individuals suffering from occipital neuralgia. Here are the key benefits:

Reduced Inflammation

An anti-inflammatory diet is rich in foods that help decrease inflammation in the body. This can directly impact the occipital nerves by reducing irritation and swelling, which are common causes of pain in occipital neuralgia.

Pain Management

By lowering inflammation, an anti-inflammatory diet can contribute to pain relief. Foods like fatty fish, leafy greens, and berries contain nutrients that have been shown to mitigate the body's inflammatory response, potentially leading to reduced pain intensity and frequency.

Improved Nerve Health

Nutrients present in anti-inflammatory foods, such as omega-3 fatty acids, vitamins, and antioxidants, support overall nerve health. These nutrients help in repairing and protecting nerve cells, which is crucial for individuals with occipital neuralgia.

Enhanced Blood Circulation

Consuming foods that promote good blood circulation ensures that vital nutrients and oxygen reach the affected areas more efficiently. Improved circulation can aid in faster recovery and reduce muscle tension around the occipital nerves.

Stress Reduction

Certain anti-inflammatory foods also possess stress-relieving properties. For instance, foods rich in magnesium, such as nuts and seeds, can help relax muscles and reduce stress, which is often a trigger for occipital neuralgia flare-ups.

Better Immune Function

A strong immune system helps to ward off infections and illnesses that may exacerbate neuralgia symptoms. An anti-inflammatory diet bolsters immune function, making the body more resilient against factors that may trigger or worsen pain.

Weight Management

Maintaining a healthy weight is essential for reducing the strain on the neck and back muscles, which can indirectly benefit those with occipital neuralgia. An anti-inflammatory diet promotes weight management by encouraging the consumption of nutrient-dense, low-calorie foods.

Reduced Reliance on Medication

Although dietary changes should complement medical treatments, adopting an anti-inflammatory diet may reduce the need for frequent medication use. This can minimize potential side effects associated with long-term medication use.

Overall Well-Being

Beyond managing pain, an anti-inflammatory diet contributes to overall well-being. It improves energy levels, enhances mood, and supports better sleep quality, all of which can positively impact the daily life of someone suffering from occipital neuralgia.

Incorporating an anti-inflammatory diet as part of a comprehensive management plan for occipital neuralgia can lead to improved symptom control and a better quality of life. Always consult with a healthcare provider or nutritionist to tailor dietary choices to individual health needs and conditions.

Disadvantages of the Diet

While an anti-inflammatory diet can provide many benefits for those with occipital neuralgia, it is important to also consider potential drawbacks.

Restrictive Nature

The anti-inflammatory diet restricts many foods that are commonly enjoyed in modern diets, such as processed and high-fat foods. This can make it challenging for some individuals to adhere to the diet long-term.

Expense

Eating a diet rich in fresh fruits, vegetables, and high-quality proteins may come at a higher cost compared to processed and packaged foods. This could be a barrier for some individuals looking to adopt an anti-inflammatory diet.

Not a One-Size-Fits-All Solution

As with any dietary change, individual results may vary. What works for one person may not work for another, and some individuals may not see significant improvements in their symptoms from adopting an anti-inflammatory diet alone. It is always important to work closely with a healthcare provider to develop a personalized treatment plan that addresses all aspects of occipital neuralgia.

Although there may be some limitations to an anti-inflammatory diet, its potential benefits make it a valuable tool in the management of occipital neuralgia. By reducing inflammation and promoting overall health, this diet can contribute to improved symptom control and a better quality of life for those living with this condition.

5-Step-by-Step Guide to Starting an Anti-Inflammatory Diet for Occipital Neuralgia

Starting a new diet can feel overwhelming, but with a clear plan in place, it can be manageable and even enjoyable. Here is a 5-step guide to help you get started on an anti-inflammatory diet for occipital neuralgia.

Step 1: Educate Yourself

Before diving into any new diet, it is essential to educate yourself on its principles and guidelines. Understanding the rationale behind the anti-inflammatory diet will help you make informed choices that can positively impact your health, particularly if you are managing occipital neuralgia.

Understand Why Certain Foods Are Restricted or Recommended

The first step in educating yourself is to grasp why certain foods are either restricted or recommended in an anti-inflammatory diet. Foods that cause inflammation often contain high levels of sugar, trans fats, and refined carbohydrates.

These can exacerbate pain and discomfort associated with conditions like occipital neuralgia. On the other hand, anti-inflammatory foods are rich in nutrients that help reduce inflammation and promote overall health. Knowing the science behind these dietary choices can enhance your commitment and adherence to the diet.

Research Recipes and Meal Plans

A practical way to prepare for your new dietary journey is by exploring recipes and meal plans tailored for an anti-inflammatory diet. This research will give you a clearer idea of what types of meals you can enjoy while adhering to the diet's guidelines.

Look for a variety of breakfast, lunch, dinner, and snack options that incorporate anti-inflammatory ingredients. Websites, cookbooks, and food blogs focused on anti-inflammatory diets can be valuable resources. Having a collection of go-to recipes will make meal planning more straightforward and enjoyable.

Consult with a Registered Dietitian

For personalized guidance, consider consulting with a registered dietitian who specializes in anti-inflammatory diets. A dietitian can assess your specific needs, preferences, and health goals to create a customized plan that works best for you.

They can also provide tips on how to transition smoothly into this new way of eating, recommend portion sizes, and suggest suitable substitutions for restricted foods. Their expertise ensures that your diet is not only effective but also balanced and nutritionally complete.

Utilize Educational Resources

Take advantage of the wealth of educational resources available to deepen your understanding of the anti-inflammatory diet. Books, online courses, webinars, and seminars led by nutrition experts can offer valuable insights and practical advice. Engaging with these resources can also keep you motivated and informed about the latest research and trends in anti-inflammatory nutrition.

By thoroughly educating yourself on the anti-inflammatory diet, you set a solid foundation for success. This preparation empowers you to make wise food choices that support your health and well-being, ultimately helping you manage occipital neuralgia more effectively.

Step 2: Eliminate Inflammatory Foods

To effectively manage occipital neuralgia through diet, it's crucial to identify and eliminate foods that can cause inflammation. Removing these offenders from your diet will help reduce pain and discomfort, contributing to overall well-being.

1. **Common Inflammatory Foods to Avoid**

    Start by familiarizing yourself with the most common inflammatory foods. These typically include:

    - Processed Foods: Items such as pre-packaged snacks, fast food, and processed meats often contain preservatives, artificial additives, and unhealthy fats that promote inflammation.
    - Sugary Snacks: Foods and beverages high in sugar, including sodas, candies, pastries, and sweetened cereals, can spike blood sugar levels and trigger inflammatory responses.
    - Refined Carbohydrates: White bread, white rice, pasta, and other refined grains lack fiber and essential nutrients, leading to rapid increases in blood sugar and subsequent inflammation.
    - Trans Fats: Found in many fried foods, margarine, and commercially baked goods, trans fats contribute significantly to inflammation and should be completely avoided.

2. **Reading Labels**

    Develop the habit of reading food labels carefully. Ingredients are listed in order of quantity, so if sugar, refined grains, or hydrogenated oils appear at the top of the list, it's best to avoid those products. Look for hidden sugars under names like high-fructose corn syrup, dextrose, and sucrose. Similarly, steer clear of items listing trans fats or partially hydrogenated oils.

3. **Opt for Whole, Unprocessed Alternatives**

Replacing inflammatory foods with whole, unprocessed alternatives is a key strategy. Focus on incorporating:

- Whole Grains: Brown rice, quinoa, barley, and whole oats are excellent substitutes for refined grains. They provide fiber, vitamins, and minerals without causing spikes in blood sugar.
- Fresh Produce: Fill your plate with a variety of colorful fruits and vegetables. These are naturally anti-inflammatory due to their high content of antioxidants, vitamins, and minerals.
- Healthy Fats: Replace trans fats with healthy fats found in olive oil, avocados, nuts, and seeds. These fats support heart health and help reduce inflammation.
- Lean Proteins: Choose lean proteins such as fish, chicken, turkey, tofu, and legumes. Fatty fish like salmon and mackerel are particularly beneficial due to their omega-3 fatty acids.

- Natural Sweeteners: If you need to satisfy a sweet tooth, opt for natural sweeteners like honey, maple syrup, or fresh fruit. Use them in moderation to keep sugar intake low.

4. **Practical Tips for Elimination**
    - Meal Prep: Prepare meals at home using fresh ingredients to control what goes into your food.
    - Shop Smart: Shop the perimeter of the grocery store where fresh produce, meats, and dairy are located. Avoid the center aisles where processed foods are typically displayed.
    - Stay Hydrated: Drink plenty of water instead of sugary drinks. Herbal teas and infused water are great options too.

By eliminating inflammatory foods and opting for whole, unprocessed alternatives, you can significantly reduce inflammation and improve your symptoms of occipital neuralgia. This step lays the groundwork for a healthier, more balanced diet that supports long-term well-being.

Step 3: Plan Balanced Meals

Creating a balanced meal plan is essential for maintaining an anti-inflammatory diet that supports overall health and helps manage occipital neuralgia. A well-structured meal plan ensures you get the right mix of proteins, healthy fats, and carbohydrates, all from anti-inflammatory sources.

Balance Proteins, Healthy Fats, and Carbohydrates

The key to a balanced meal is incorporating essential macronutrients—proteins, fats, and carbohydrates—in appropriate proportions. Here's how you can achieve this:

- *Proteins*: Proteins are vital for muscle repair, immune function, and overall body maintenance. Opt for lean protein sources such as fish (especially those rich in omega-3 fatty acids like salmon and mackerel), poultry, beans, lentils, tofu, and tempeh. These proteins support muscle health and provide anti-inflammatory benefits.
- *Healthy Fats*: Healthy fats help reduce inflammation and support brain and heart health. Integrate sources like olive oil, avocados, nuts (almonds, walnuts), seeds (chia, flax), and fatty fish into your meals. These fats also enhance the absorption of fat-soluble vitamins.
- *Carbohydrates*: Carbohydrates provide the energy needed for daily activities. Choose complex carbohydrates from whole grains, such as quinoa, brown rice, barley, and whole oats. These sources are high in fiber, which aids digestion and helps maintain stable blood sugar levels, thus reducing inflammation.

Aim for Colorful Plates

A colorful plate is often a signal of a nutritious and well-balanced meal. Different colors in fruits and vegetables typically indicate various essential nutrients and antioxidants:

- ***Red and Purple***: Foods like tomatoes, berries, and beets are rich in antioxidants such as lycopene and anthocyanins, which combat oxidative stress and reduce inflammation.
- ***Green***: Leafy greens like spinach, kale, and broccoli are packed with vitamins C, E, and K, along with fiber and antioxidants that support overall health and reduce inflammation.
- ***Orange and Yellow***: Carrots, sweet potatoes, and bell peppers contain beta-carotene and vitamin C, both powerful antioxidants that help decrease inflammation.
- ***White and Brown***: Garlic, onions, and mushrooms offer anti-inflammatory compounds and support the immune system.

Create a Weekly Meal Plan

Structuring a weekly meal plan ensures you have a diverse intake of nutrients and helps prevent mealtime stress. Here's a practical approach:

- ***Breakfast***: Start your day with a mix of complex carbs, proteins, and healthy fats. For example, oatmeal topped with chia seeds, fresh berries, and a drizzle of honey or a smoothie made with spinach, avocado, almond milk, and a scoop of protein powder.
- ***Lunch***: Aim for a hearty salad or grain bowl. Combine leafy greens with quinoa, grilled chicken or chickpeas,

avocado slices, and a variety of colorful vegetables. Dress with olive oil and lemon juice.
- **Dinner**: Focus on lean proteins and cooked vegetables. A typical meal could include baked salmon with a side of roasted Brussels sprouts and sweet potato wedges.
- **Snacks**: Keep snacks simple and nutritious. Consider options like a handful of nuts, fresh fruit, hummus with carrot sticks, or yogurt with flaxseeds.

Practical Tips for Balanced Meal Planning

- *Prep Ahead*: Spend some time each week prepping ingredients. Cook batches of whole grains and proteins that you can mix and match throughout the week.
- *Variety Is Key*: Rotate different proteins, vegetables, and whole grains to keep meals interesting and nutritionally diverse.
- *Listen to Your Body*: Pay attention to how different foods make you feel. Adjust your meal plan based on what best supports your energy levels and reduces symptoms.

By carefully planning balanced meals that incorporate a variety of anti-inflammatory ingredients, you can support your body's nutritional needs and help alleviate the symptoms of occipital neuralgia. This thoughtful approach to eating fosters long-term health and well-being.

Step 4: Stay Hydrated

Staying properly hydrated is a fundamental aspect of maintaining overall health and managing inflammation, which is crucial for relieving symptoms of occipital neuralgia. Here are some detailed strategies to keep your hydration on track:

Drink Plenty of Water

Aim to drink at least 8 glasses (about 2 liters) of water each day, though individual needs may vary based on factors such as activity level, climate, and overall health. Water plays a key role in various bodily functions, including nutrient transport, digestion, and temperature regulation. Staying well-hydrated helps flush out toxins that can contribute to inflammation and keeps your joints and muscles functioning smoothly.

Incorporate Herbal Teas

Herbal teas are an excellent way to boost your hydration while also providing additional health benefits. Teas made from ginger, turmeric, chamomile, and green tea have anti-inflammatory properties and can be soothing. They are typically caffeine-free, which makes them a good choice for hydration without the diuretic effects of caffeinated beverages.

Eat Water-Rich Fruits and Vegetables

Incorporate water-rich fruits and vegetables into your diet to supplement your fluid intake:

- *Cucumber*: Composed of about 95% water, cucumbers are incredibly hydrating and can be easily added to salads, sandwiches, or enjoyed as a snack.
- *Watermelon*: With a water content of about 92%, watermelon is not only refreshing but also rich in vitamins A and C, which have anti-inflammatory properties.
- *Other Options*: Tomatoes, oranges, strawberries, and bell peppers are also high in water content and provide essential nutrients and antioxidants.

Practical Tips for Staying Hydrated

- *Carry a Water Bottle*: Keep a reusable water bottle with you throughout the day to remind yourself to drink regularly.
- *Set Reminders*: Use phone alarms or apps to set reminders to drink water at regular intervals.
- *Infuse Your Water*: Add slices of lemon, lime, cucumber, or fresh herbs like mint to your water to enhance its flavor and make it more enjoyable to drink.

Step 5: Monitor and Adjust

Keeping track of your dietary habits and their effects on your symptoms is a crucial step in managing occipital neuralgia through an anti-inflammatory diet. Here's how to effectively monitor and adjust your eating plan:

Keep a Food Diary

Maintain a detailed food diary to log everything you eat and drink. Include the following information:

- *Daily Food Intake*: Write down all meals, snacks, and beverages consumed throughout the day.
- *Portion Sizes*: Record approximate portion sizes to help identify potential issues with overeating or under-eating certain foods.
- *Symptoms*: Note any symptoms you experience, such as pain flare-ups, headaches, or improvements in discomfort levels.
- *Time of Day*: Include the times you ate and experienced symptoms to identify patterns.

Analyze Patterns

Review your food diary regularly to identify any correlations between specific foods and your symptoms. Look for:

- *Improvement Trends*: Determine which anti-inflammatory foods are associated with reduced

pain and inflammation, and continue to emphasize these in your diet.
- *Trigger Foods*: Identify any foods that seem to trigger symptoms or exacerbate pain. Gradually eliminate or reduce these items from your diet.

Adjust Your Diet Accordingly

Based on your analysis, make informed adjustments to your meal plans:

- *Emphasize Anti-Inflammatory Foods*: Increase the frequency and portions of foods that help reduce inflammation and improve symptoms.
- *Modify Recipes*: Adapt your favorite recipes to include more anti-inflammatory ingredients and avoid known triggers.
- *Experiment with New Foods*: Introduce new anti-inflammatory foods and monitor their effects on your symptoms.

Consult Professionals

Consider consulting with a registered dietitian or healthcare provider, especially if you're experiencing significant difficulties in identifying triggers or managing symptoms. They can provide tailored advice and support to fine-tune your diet.

Practical Tips for Monitoring and Adjusting

- *Use Apps*: There are several food diary apps available that can make tracking easier and more efficient.
- *Stay Consistent*: Aim to log your food and symptoms daily for the most accurate insights.
- *Be Patient*: It may take time to determine the full impact of dietary changes on your symptoms, so maintain patience and consistency in your efforts.

By staying hydrated and meticulously monitoring your diet, you can make informed adjustments that support your health and help manage the symptoms of occipital neuralgia more effectively. This proactive approach ensures that your anti-inflammatory diet is personalized and responsive to your body's needs.

Foods to Eat

While there is no cure for occipital neuralgia, following an anti-inflammatory diet can help to lessen symptoms and improve your quality of life. The focus of an anti-inflammatory diet is on foods that reduce inflammation, which can alleviate pain and discomfort associated with occipital neuralgia. Here are the key food groups to emphasize

Fruits

Fruits are rich in antioxidants, vitamins, and fiber, all of which play a role in reducing inflammation.

- *Berries*: Blueberries, strawberries, raspberries, and blackberries are packed with antioxidants like anthocyanins, which help combat inflammation.
- *Citrus Fruits*: Oranges, lemons, limes, and grapefruits provide vitamin C and flavonoids, both known for their anti-inflammatory properties.
- *Other Fruits*: Apples, cherries, and pineapples also contribute valuable antioxidants and nutrients.

Vegetables

Vegetables are essential for their high vitamin, mineral, and phytochemical content, all contributing to reduced inflammation.

- *Leafy Greens*: Spinach, kale, Swiss chard, and collard greens are rich in vitamins A, C, K, and folate, and contain anti-inflammatory compounds.
- *Cruciferous Vegetables*: Broccoli, Brussels sprouts, cauliflower, and cabbage are high in antioxidants and fiber.
- *Colorful Vegetables*: Carrots, bell peppers, squash, and sweet potatoes offer a variety of antioxidants, vitamins, and minerals.

Whole Grains

Whole grains are a good source of fiber, which supports a healthy gut and helps reduce inflammation.

- *Quinoa*: A complete protein that is high in fiber and various essential nutrients.
- *Brown Rice*: Provides fiber and magnesium, promoting anti-inflammatory effects.
- *Oats*: High in beta-glucans, which have been shown to reduce inflammation.

Lean Protein

Protein is essential for muscle repair and overall health, and choosing lean sources helps minimize inflammation.

- *Fish*: Fatty fish such as salmon, mackerel, sardines, and trout are rich in omega-3 fatty acids, which are potent anti-inflammatories.
- *Poultry*: Chicken and turkey are excellent lean protein sources without added fats.
- *Plant-Based Proteins*: Lentils, chickpeas, beans, tofu, and tempeh offer plant-based protein along with fiber and other beneficial nutrients.

Healthy Fats

Healthy fats are crucial for reducing inflammation and supporting heart and brain health.

- **Olive Oil**: Extra virgin olive oil is rich in monounsaturated fats and contains oleocanthal, which has anti-inflammatory effects similar to ibuprofen.
- **Avocados**: Packed with monounsaturated fats, fiber, and antioxidants.
- **Nuts and Seeds**: Almonds, walnuts, chia seeds, and flax seeds provide healthy fats, fiber, and omega-3 fatty acids.

Hydrating Foods

Proper hydration is vital for reducing inflammation and maintaining overall health.

- **Cucumber**: High water content and anti-inflammatory properties.
- **Watermelon**: Refreshing and hydrating, with vitamins A and C.
- **Celery**: Contains antioxidants and anti-inflammatory compounds while providing hydration.

By emphasizing these anti-inflammatory foods in your diet, you can help reduce the symptoms of occipital neuralgia and enhance your overall quality of life.

Foods to Avoid

In addition to eating anti-inflammatory foods, it's crucial to avoid foods that can trigger or worsen inflammation. While individual triggers can vary, there are some common culprits that are generally known to promote inflammation and exacerbate symptoms of occipital neuralgia.

Processed Foods

Processed foods often contain unhealthy fats, additives, and preservatives that can contribute to inflammation.

- ***Fast Food***: Burgers, fries, and other fast food items are typically high in trans fats and refined carbohydrates.
- ***Packaged Snacks***: Chips, crackers, and sugary snacks often contain preservatives, artificial flavors, and unhealthy oils.

Sugary Foods and Beverages

High sugar intake can lead to spikes in blood sugar and insulin levels, which can trigger inflammatory responses.

- ***Sugary Snacks***: Candies, pastries, cookies, and cakes are loaded with sugars that contribute to inflammation.
- ***Sweetened Beverages***: Sodas, energy drinks, and sweetened tea or coffee drinks can contain large amounts of added sugars.

Refined Carbohydrates

Refined carbohydrates lack fiber and essential nutrients, leading to rapid increases in blood sugar and subsequent inflammation.

- ***White Bread and Pasta***: Made from refined flour, these products can spike blood sugar levels.
- ***White Rice***: Unlike brown rice, white rice has had its fibrous outer layer removed, making it less nutritious.

Trans Fats

Trans fats are known to be highly inflammatory and are often found in fried and commercially baked goods.

- ***Fried Foods***: French fries, fried chicken, and doughnuts are cooked in oils containing trans fats.
- ***Commercial Baked Goods***: Cookies, cakes, and pastries often contain partially hydrogenated oils.

Red and Processed Meats

Red and processed meats can be high in saturated fats and advanced glycation end products (AGEs), which promote inflammation.

- ***Red Meat***: Beef, pork, and lamb should be consumed in moderation.
- ***Processed Meats***: Sausages, bacon, and deli meats often contain additives and preservatives that can trigger inflammation.

Dairy Products

Some people may find that dairy products worsen their inflammation due to lactose intolerance or sensitivity to casein.

- *Whole Milk and Cream*: High in saturated fats, which can contribute to inflammation.
- *Cheese and Butter*: This can be difficult to digest for some individuals, potentially worsening inflammation.

Alcohol

Excessive alcohol consumption can lead to increased inflammatory markers in the body.

- *Beer and Spirits*: High alcohol content can exacerbate inflammation.
- *Cocktails*: Often include sugary mixers that further contribute to inflammatory responses.

Practical Tips for Avoiding Inflammatory Foods

- *Read Labels*: Always check food labels for hidden sugars, trans fats, and additives.
- *Cook at Home*: Preparing meals at home allows you to control the ingredients and avoid hidden inflammatory substances.
- *Opt for Alternatives*: Look for healthier alternatives to your favorite snacks and meals. For example, choose

whole grain bread instead of white bread, and opt for grilled fish instead of fried chicken.

- ***Moderation is Key***: If you can't completely eliminate certain foods, aim to reduce their consumption and balance them with anti-inflammatory foods.

By identifying and avoiding these common inflammatory foods, you can help manage the symptoms of occipital neuralgia more effectively and improve your overall health.

7-Day Sample Meal Plan

Here's a balanced, anti-inflammatory meal plan that incorporates the provided recipes and adheres to the food restrictions. This plan ensures variety and nutritional balance to help manage occipital neuralgia symptoms.

Day 1

Breakfast:

- Overnight oats with chia seeds, blueberries, and almond milk

Lunch:

- Cheddar Turkey Deviled Eggs
- Mixed green salad with olive oil and lemon dressing

Snack:

- Apple slices with almond butter

Dinner:

- Ginger Chicken Stir Fry
- Steamed brown rice

Day 2

Breakfast:

- Smoothie with spinach, banana, flaxseed, and unsweetened almond milk

Lunch:

- Slow Cooker Dairy-Free Buttered Chicken
- Quinoa and steamed broccoli

Snack:

- Carrot sticks with hummus

Dinner:

- Baked Sea Bass with Lemon Dressing
- Roasted Brussels sprouts and sweet potato wedges

Day 3

Breakfast:

- Greek yogurt with honey, walnuts, and fresh berries

Lunch:

- Cauliflower Rice with Chicken and Broccoli

Snack:

- Handful of mixed nuts (almonds, walnuts)

Dinner:

- Salmon Fillet with Lemon and Garlic
- Sautéed spinach and quinoa

Day 4

Breakfast:

- Scrambled eggs with spinach and tomatoes

Lunch:

- Grilled Tuna
- Mixed greens with cucumber and olive oil dressing

Snack:

- Fresh orange or grapefruit segments

Dinner:

- Cod Pea Curry
- Brown rice

Day 5

Breakfast:

- Whole grain toast with avocado and a poached egg

Lunch:

- Baked Flounder
- Steamed asparagus and wild rice

Snack:

- Celery sticks with almond butter

Dinner:

- Lemon-Baked Salmon
- Roasted root vegetables (carrots, parsnips, sweet potatoes)

Day 6

Breakfast:

- Chia pudding with coconut milk, topped with sliced strawberries and almonds

Lunch:

- Roasted Bone Broth
- Side salad with kale, cherry tomatoes, and olive oil

Snack:

- Sliced bell peppers with guacamole

Dinner:

- Baked Salmon
- Steamed green beans and quinoa

Day 7

Breakfast:

- Smoothie bowl with blended spinach, banana, almond milk, topped with flaxseeds and fresh fruit

Lunch:

- Lentil soup with carrots, celery, and kale

Snack:

- Fresh pineapple slices

Dinner:

- Herb-roasted chicken breast
- Mixed roasted vegetables (zucchini, bell peppers, onions)
- Brown rice

This meal plan incorporates a variety of anti-inflammatory foods, lean proteins, whole grains, and healthy fats to help reduce inflammation and manage symptoms of occipital neuralgia effectively.

Sample Recipes

We have included some sample recipes for each meal to help give you an idea of how these meals can be prepared and cooked.

Baked Flounder

Ingredients:

- 1 lb. flounder, fileted
- 1/4 tsp. salt
- 1 cup halved red grapes
- 1 tbsp. extra-virgin olive oil
- 2 tbsp. parsley, chopped finely
- 1 tbsp. lemon juice
- 1 cup almonds, chopped and toasted
- freshly ground black pepper, to taste

Instructions:

1. Preheat the oven to 375°F.
2. Place fish on a sheet tray. Season with olive oil, salt, and pepper.
3. Combine the almonds, grapes, lemon juice, parsley, 1-1/2 tsp. of olive oil, 1/8 tsp of salt, and black pepper in a bowl.
4. Bake the fish for about 3 minutes.
5. Flip the fish and return it to the oven.
6. Bake for another 3 minutes, or until the fish is starting to flake, while the center is still translucent. Don't overcook.
7. Serve immediately, topped with the grape mixture.

Baked Salmon

Ingredients:

- 2 salmon filets
- 6 cups of fresh spinach
- 2 tsp. coconut oil
- 1/4 tsp. garlic powder
- 1/4 tsp. turmeric
- 3 large cloves of garlic
- lemon juice
- salt
- pepper

Instructions:

1. Preheat the oven to 400°F.
2. Line a baking dish with parchment paper.
3. Marinate salmon filets in lemon juice, coconut oil, garlic powder, turmeric, salt, and pepper.
4. Let it sit for a few minutes. This may also be done the night before to help the juices and flavor get into the salmon.
5. Once the oven is ready, bake salmon for 15 minutes.
6. Cook some of the garlic in a pan with coconut oil.
7. Add spinach and cook until ready. Season with salt and pepper to taste.
8. Take salmon out of the oven and put spinach beside it.
9. Serve and enjoy.

Lemon-Baked Salmon

Ingredients:

- 2 pcs. lemons, thinly sliced
- 3 lbs. salmon filet
- kosher salt
- black pepper, freshly ground
- 6 tbsp. butter, melted, 6 tbsp.
- 2 tbsp. honey
- 3 cloves garlic, minced
- 1 tsp. thyme leaves, chopped
- 1 tsp. dried oregano
- fresh parsley, chopped, for garnish

Instructions:

1. Preheat the oven to 350°F.
2. Line a rimmed baking sheet with foil. Grease with cooking oil spray.
3. Lay lemon slices on the center of the foil.
4. Season salmon filets on both sides with kosher salt and freshly ground black pepper.
5. Place the filet on top of the lemon slices.
6. Whisk together oregano, thyme, garlic, honey, and butter in a small bowl.
7. Pour the mixture over the salmon filet.
8. Fold the foil up and around the salmon to form a packet.

9. Bake for 25 minutes or until the salmon is cooked through.
10. Switch to broil and continue cooking for 2 more minutes.
11. Garnish with chopped fresh parsley and serve hot.

Cod Pea Curry

Instructions:

- 1 onion, sliced
- 1 tbsp. extra-virgin olive oil
- 1 tsp. cumin
- 1 tsp. mustard powder
- 1/2 tsp. turmeric
- 1 tbsp. fresh ginger, minced
- 1 tsp. garlic, minced
- a pinch of salt
- freshly ground black pepper
- 2 tbsp. cilantro, chopped finely
- 1 medium head cauliflower, broken into small florets, approximately half-inch pieces
- 1-lb. cod, cut into about half an inch cube,
- 2 cups peas, fresh or frozen
- 4 cups spinach

Instructions:

1. Heat a large heavy-bottomed stock pot over low heat.
2. Add the olive oil and onion and cook until translucent, stirring often about 5 minutes.
3. Add the garlic, ginger, mustard powder, cumin, salt, turmeric, and black pepper. Cook for 1 more minute, stirring constantly.
4. Add the cilantro and 4-1/2 cups of water. Leave to boil.

5. Then, reduce heat to simmer for about 10 minutes.
6. Toss in the cauliflower. Leave to simmer for 2 more minutes.
7. Add in the peas, cod, and spinach. Stir and cover. Leave to simmer for another 4 minutes.
8. Serve and enjoy immediately.

Grilled Tuna

Ingredients:

- tuna
- 4 tbsp. lemon juice
- 2 cloves garlic, minced
- salt
- pepper

Instructions:

1. Marinate tuna with garlic and lemon juice.
2. Season with salt and pepper.
3. Grill for 8-10 minutes.
4. Add more fresh ground pepper upon serving.
5. Serve and enjoy while hot.

Baked Sea Bass and Lemon Dressing

Ingredients:

- 4 100g sea bass filets
- 3 tbsp. extra-virgin olive oil
- 2 tbsp. small capers
- 1 grated lemon zest
- 2 tbsp. flat-leaf parsley, chopped
- 2 tsp. gluten-free Dijon mustard

Instructions:

1. Using a small mixing bowl, make a salad dressing by mixing the lemon juice, zest, mustard, capers, seasonings, and water. Do not include the parsley.
2. Preheat the oven to 200°C.
3. Line the baking tray with parchment paper and place the fish filets.
4. Brush the skin of the fish with some olive oil and sprinkle it with salt.
5. Bake for 7-9 minutes or until the flesh flakes when tested with a fork or a knife.
6. Arrange the fish on a large serving plate and garnish with extra parsley leaves.

Roasted Bone Broth

Ingredients:

- 4 lbs. beef bones, such as marrow bones or bones with a layer of meat
- 1 leek, cut into 2-inch pieces
- 2 carrots, cut into 2-inch pieces
- 1 garlic head, halved
- 1 onion, quartered
- 2 tbsp. black peppercorns
- 2 bay leaves
- 1 tbsp. cider vinegar
- 2 celery stalks, cut into 2-inch pieces

Instructions:

1. Preheat the oven to about 450°F.
2. On a rimmed baking sheet or a roasting pan, put the bones, onion, garlic, carrots, and leek. Put this in the oven to roast for about 20 minutes.
3. Take it out of the oven to toss. Roast for about 20 minutes more or until the contents are browned deeply.
4. Pour water into a large stockpot, about 12 cups or so.
5. Add celery, bay leaves, vinegar, and peppercorns.
6. Transfer all the roasted contents to the pot, including the juice, if any.
7. If needed, add more water. Make sure that everything is covered. Cover the pan with the lid.

8. Bring it to a gentle boil.
9. Then, reduce heat to a low simmer and slightly open the lid while you cook. From time to time, skim the foam and excess fat floating in the broth.
10. Leave to simmer for a while to get a better broth taste. Add water if needed.
11. Once done, move the pot away from the heat. Separate solids from the broth using a sieve. Boiled vegetables and bones may be discarded.
12. Allow to cool down until it's barely warm, before refrigerating.
13. When serving, make sure to remove the hardened fat on top of the broth before heating.

Salmon Fillet with Lemon and Garlic

Ingredients:

- 1 large salmon filet
- 1/4 cup fresh cilantro leaves, chopped roughly
- 4 cloves of garlic, minced
- 1 lemon
- Kosher salt, to taste
- black pepper, to taste
- Optional: 1 tbsp. butter

Instructions:

1. Preheat the oven or grill to 400°F.
2. Line a baking sheet with foil. Don't grease it.
3. Place salmon on the foil, skin side down.
4. Season the filet by squeezing lemon over it. Then, evenly sprinkle the filet with cilantro, garlic, salt, and pepper over the top.
5. Optional: Thinly slice butter and place pieces evenly over the top of the salmon.
6. For the grill, cook salmon for about 15 minutes.
7. For the oven, cook salmon for about 7 minutes, depending on its thickness.
8. Turn the oven up to broil and continue to cook for an additional 5-7 minutes, until the top is crispy.

9. Remove the salmon from the oven or grill and slide a flat spatula in between the salmon and the skin. Leave the skin to stick to the foil.
10. Serve while hot.

Cauliflower Rice with Chicken and Broccoli

Ingredients:

- 1 broccoli head
- 1 cauliflower head
- 2 chicken breasts, boneless and skinless
- 1 tbsp. olive oil
- salt
- pepper

Instructions:

1. Preheat the oven to 350°F.
2. Cut the broccoli into small florets.
3. Remove the core from the cauliflower and chop it into small pieces.
4. In a food processor, pulse the cauliflower until it resembles rice.
5. In a baking dish, combine broccoli, cauliflower rice, chicken, and olive oil. Season with salt and pepper.
6. Bake for 20-25 minutes, or until the chicken is cooked through.

Slow Cooker Dairy-Free Buttered Chicken

Ingredients:

- 2 lbs. boneless and skinless chicken breast, chopped into chunks
- 15 oz. can of full-fat coconut milk
- 15 oz. can of tomato sauce
- 2 tbsp. lemon juice
- 1 cinnamon stick
- 2 tbsp. coconut oil
- 1 tsp. sea salt
- 1 pc. chopped yellow onion
- 5 cloves minced garlic
- 1 tsp chili powder
- 1/2 tsp. cayenne powder
- 1 in. knob ginger, chopped
- 2 tsp. ground turmeric
- 1 tbsp. garam masala
- 1 tbsp. cumin
- 1/2 ground pepper
- 1/2 tsp. ground cinnamon

Instructions:

1. Preheat the skillet and add oil.
2. Sauté onion and garlic for 5 minutes.

3. Add turmeric, garam masala, ginger, salt, pepper, chili powder, cayenne, and cinnamon. Toss to combine all spices. Cook for 1-2 minutes.
4. Transfer the mixture to the slow cooker.
5. Add chicken, coconut milk, lemon juice, tomato sauce, and cinnamon. Cover and cook for 2-3 hours over high heat.
6. Serve hot and garnish with fresh cilantro and some lime juice.

Ginger Chicken Stir Fry

Ingredients:

Stir-fry mix:

- 1 lb. cooked chicken, dark or light meat
- 4 cups cremini mushrooms, sliced
- 4 cups purple cabbage, sliced
- 2 cups carrots
- 1/2 cup green onions, cut slanted
- 3 cups cauliflower florets
- 1 handful of enoki mushrooms
- 2 tbsp. avocado oil
- 1 package of rice noodles, cook according to instructions

Stir-fry sauce:

- 4 cloves minced garlic
- 1/4 cup honey
- 1/4 tsp. grated ginger
- 1/4 cup rice wine vinegar
- 1 cup chicken stock
- 1 tbsp. avocado oil

Instructions:

To make the stir-fry sauce:

1. Cook garlic with oil on low to medium heat

2. Once the garlic is browned, add in the honey. Let the sauce bubble for a moment.
3. Add in the vinegar and cover with a lid.
4. Pour in the chicken stock. Leave to boil until reduced by half.
5. Season with salt and pepper.

To make the stir-fry mix:

1. Heat the oil in a large wok. Cook the vegetables, adding them one by one according to the degree of hardness.
2. Once the vegetables are well-caramelized, add in the chicken and noodles and heat through.
3. Pour in the stir-fry sauce and mix well.
4. Garnish with green onions.

Cheddar Turkey Deviled Egg

Ingredients:

- 6 large organic eggs
- 2 slices of nitrate-free turkey bacon
- 1/4 cup low-fat cheddar cheese, shredded OR grated
- 3 tbsp. light mayonnaise
- 1 tsp. white wine vinegar
- 1/2 tsp. chives, chopped
- 1/8 tsp. ground black pepper
- 1/8 tsp. salt

Instructions:

1. Place the eggs in a large pot or saucepan.
2. Pour cold water into the pot or pan until the water is covering the eggs by 1-1/2 inches.
3. Bring the water to a boil over high heat.
4. Once it has boiled, remove it from the stove.
5. Cover and let it stand for 12 to 15 minutes.
6. When it has cooled down, peel off the egg's shells.
7. Fry the bacon slices using medium-high heat in a non-stick skillet until bacon slices have become crispy but not burnt.
8. Transfer fried bacon into paper towels to drain off the excess oil.
9. Once it has cooled down, break down the bacon into small bits. Set aside.

10. Cut the hard-boiled eggs in half, lengthwise.
11. Gently carve out the egg yolks into a medium-sized bowl.
12. Arrange the hollowed-out egg halves in a flat container.
13. Add the rest of the ingredients to the bowl with the yolk.
14. Stir well until the texture has become smooth.
15. Transfer the mixture into a piping bag or resealable bag with a trimmed corner.
16. Pipe the yolk mixture back into the egg halves.
17. Sprinkle each filled egg halves with bacon bits.
18. Serve immediately or after it has been chilled for at least half an hour.

Conclusion

Thank you for taking the time to read our comprehensive guide on managing occipital neuralgia through diet. We hope this resource has provided you with valuable insights and practical strategies to help alleviate and manage the symptoms associated with this condition.

Throughout this guide, we have explored the critical role that diet can play in managing occipital neuralgia. By making mindful dietary choices, focusing on anti-inflammatory foods, and avoiding known triggers, you can take significant steps toward reducing the frequency and intensity of your headaches.

Remember that a balanced diet rich in nutrients is crucial for overall health and well-being, particularly when dealing with chronic pain conditions like occipital neuralgia. Anti-inflammatory foods such as fatty fish, leafy greens, berries, and nuts can help reduce inflammation and potentially ease the pressure on the occipital nerves.

Staying well-hydrated is paramount; dehydration can trigger headaches and worsen symptoms, so make sure to drink plenty of water throughout the day. Avoiding common dietary triggers like processed foods, caffeine, and alcohol is also essential.

Each person's triggers can vary, so it's important to pay attention to your body's responses and adjust your diet accordingly. Foods high in magnesium, vitamin B12, and omega-3 fatty acids can be particularly beneficial in managing occipital neuralgia, supporting nerve health, and reducing inflammation.

Managing occipital neuralgia is a journey, and every step you take toward understanding and controlling your diet contributes to your overall health. It's essential to remain patient and persistent, as changes in diet may take some time to manifest noticeable improvements.

Keeping a food diary can be incredibly helpful. Tracking what you eat and how you feel can help identify patterns and specific food triggers, providing invaluable personal insight for making informed dietary choices. Always discuss any significant dietary changes with your healthcare provider, especially if you have other medical conditions or are taking medication.

They can provide personalized advice and ensure your diet supports your overall health. Nutritional science is continually evolving, so stay updated with the latest research and recommendations to ensure your diet remains optimal for managing occipital neuralgia.

Finally, consider joining support communities. Connecting with others who have occipital neuralgia can provide emotional support and practical tips. Many online communities offer shared experiences and encouragement, which can be incredibly beneficial.

Your dedication to exploring dietary changes as a means to manage occipital neuralgia demonstrates a proactive approach to your health. Remember, while diet can play a pivotal role, it is just one piece of the puzzle. A holistic approach, combining diet, exercise, stress management, and medical care, will yield the best results.

By understanding your body and making thoughtful dietary choices, you have the power to influence your health positively. Keep pushing forward, stay curious, and most importantly, be kind to yourself during this journey. Your efforts are not in vain, and every small change brings you closer to a more comfortable and healthier life.

Thank you once again for reading this guide. We hope it has inspired you to take control of your diet and, consequently, your occipital neuralgia symptoms. Remember, you're not alone, and with determination and the right tools, you can manage your condition effectively.

FAQs

Can changing my diet really help manage occipital neuralgia?

Yes, dietary changes can play a significant role in managing occipital neuralgia. By incorporating anti-inflammatory foods, staying well-hydrated, and avoiding known triggers, you can potentially reduce the frequency and intensity of your headaches. However, it's important to remember that diet is just one aspect of a comprehensive treatment plan.

What are some anti-inflammatory foods that can help with occipital neuralgia?

Anti-inflammatory foods that may help include fatty fish (like salmon and mackerel), leafy greens (such as spinach and kale), berries (like blueberries and strawberries), nuts, and seeds. These foods contain nutrients that help reduce inflammation and support overall nerve health.

Are there specific foods or beverages I should avoid?

Common dietary triggers for occipital neuralgia include processed foods, caffeine, alcohol, and foods high in sugar or artificial additives. However, triggers can vary from person to person. Keeping a food diary to track what you eat and how you feel can help identify your specific triggers.

How does hydration affect occipital neuralgia symptoms?

Staying well-hydrated is crucial because dehydration can lead to headaches and worsen occipital neuralgia symptoms. Drinking plenty of water throughout the day helps maintain overall health and can potentially reduce headache frequency and severity.

Can supplements help manage occipital neuralgia?

Certain supplements, such as magnesium, vitamin B12, and omega-3 fatty acids, may support nerve health and reduce inflammation. Before starting any new supplements, it's essential to consult with a healthcare provider to ensure they are suitable for your specific needs and won't interfere with any medications you're taking.

How long will it take to see improvements after changing my diet?

The time it takes to see improvements can vary from person to person. Dietary changes may take several weeks to months to manifest noticeable differences in symptom management. Patience and consistency are key. It's also important to combine dietary changes with other treatments and lifestyle adjustments for optimal results.

Should I consult a healthcare provider before making dietary changes?

Absolutely. Consulting with a healthcare provider or a registered dietitian is important before making significant dietary changes, especially if you have other medical conditions or are taking medications. They can provide personalized advice and help create a balanced and effective diet plan tailored to your needs.

References and Helpful Links

Da Silva De Magalhães, M. J., & Nunes, B. L. (2018). Neurectomy of C2 for the treatment of occipital neuralgia: case report. Arquivos Brasileiros De Neurocirurgia, 39(01), 046–048.
https://doi.org/10.1055/s-0037-1618598

Diet therapy for trigeminal neuralgia. (2022, September 23). Spine and Pain Clinics of North America.
https://www.sapnamed.com/blog/diet-therapy-for-trigeminal-neuralgia/
Therapy For Trigeminal Neuralgia – SAPNA Pain Management Blog. (2019, February 4). Spine and Pain Clinics of North America.
https://www.sapnamed.com/blog/diet-therapy-for-trigeminal-neuralgia/.

How to Treat Occipital Neuralgia – 21 of the Best Methods – Pain Doctor. (n.d.). Retrieved September 28, 2022, from
https://paindoctor.com/how-to-treat-occipital-neuralgia/.

All disorders. (n.d.). National Institute of Neurological Disorders and Stroke.
https://www.ninds.nih.gov/health-information/disorders/occipital-neuralgia.

BackPainSleep. (2022, September 29). Occipital neuralgia treatment at home: 3 easy methods. Back Pain Sleep.
https://backpainsleep.com/how-to-treat-occipital-neuralgia-at-home/

Vandergriendt, C. (2023, December 1). Can vitamins and supplements prevent occipital neuralgia headaches? Healthline. https://www.healthline.com/health/headache/vitamins-for-occipital-neuralgia

Occipital Neuralgia: A Beginner's Guide and Overview to Managing the Condition Through Diet, With Sample Curated Recipes - Kindle edition by Marshwell, Patrick . Health, Fitness & Dieting Kindle eBooks @ Amazon.com. (n.d.). https://www.amazon.com/Occipital-Neuralgia-Beginners-Overview-Condition-ebook/dp/B0BF9CS2W9#:~:text=Diet%20and%20nutrition%20can%20also,to%20reduce%20inflammation%20and%20pain.

Meyler, Z., DO. (n.d.). Occipital neuralgia: What it is and how to treat it. Spine-health. https://www.spine-health.com/blog/occipital-neuralgia-what-it-and-how-treat-it#:~:text=You%20may%20find%20relief%20through,inflammation%20and%20reduce%20the%20pain.

www.ingramcontent.com/pod-product-compliance
Lightning Source LLC
LaVergne TN
LVHW010428070526
838199LV00066B/5963